5BX

PLAN
FOR PHYSICAL FITNESS

FOREWORD

In preparing a foreword for this new edition of the 5BX Plan, I rediscovered its many values. Although it was developed over twenty years ago, the Five Basic Exercises are still remarkably well suited to meet today's needs. The 5BX Plan attracts and will continue to attract people interested in improving their physical condition because of its *simplicity* (five basic exercises that are easy to follow), its *effectiveness* (a program that progresses towards its goals) and, foremost, its *briefness* (each exercise session only takes 11 minutes). Like all complete and balanced exercise programs, this book describes the precautions that should be taken in following the 5BX Plan. This scientifically designed approach can help almost anyone to reach physical fitness.

Richard Chevalier
Physical Education Specialist

CAUTION

Before You Start...

If you have any doubt as to your capability to undertake this program, see your *medical adviser*.

You should not perform fast, vigorous, or highly competitive physical activity without gradually developing and continuously maintaining an adequate level of physical fitness, particularly if you are over the age of 30.

For Whom?

This exercise program has been designed for males of varying age groups.

A similar exercise program for females has been published under the title "XBX Plan for Physical Fitness," and may be purchased from the Canadian Government Publishing Center or a bookstore.

5BX Plan

Here is a new scientifically designed approach to Physical Fitness which can develop an adequate level of reserve energy needed for vigorous positive well-being and zestful living. This plan enables you to get fit:

By yourself

At home

In your spare time

At your own rate of progress

Without discomfort and

in only 11 minutes a day.

5BX *means*
FIVE BASIC EXERCISES

The 5BX Plan is unique:

SIMPLE because it is easy to do, easy to follow.

PROGRESSIVE because you can develop your own personal fitness at your own rate, to your required level, without getting stiff or sore muscles.

BALANCED because you condition your muscles, your heart and lungs harmoniously for your daily needs.

COMPLETE because the principles of muscle and organic development are applied simultaneously and progressively.

SELF-MEASURING because it gives you clear cut "targets for fitness" for your age and body build, along with graduated standards for checking your progress.

CONVENIENT because you can do these exercises any place at your convenience, without gadgets.

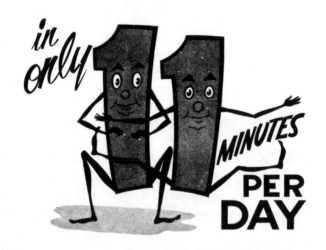

Research has demonstrated that the 5BX Plan will:

Increase the strength of the important muscle groups needed in everyday living.

Increase the ability of muscles used in essential body movements to function efficiently for long periods of time.

Increase the speed response of the important muscles of the body.

Keep the important muscles and joints of the body supple and flexible.

Improve the efficiency and capacity of the heart, lungs and other body organs.

Increase the capacity for physical exertion.

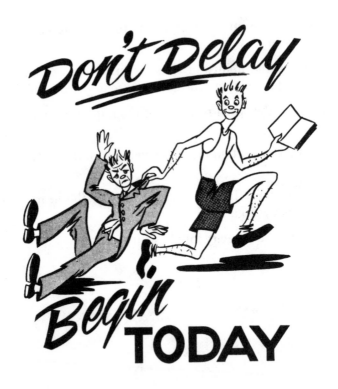

Why should you be so concerned about physical fitness?

Mechanization, automation, and work-saving devices to make life easy are depriving us of desirable physical activity. Canadians, as a result, are in danger of deteriorating physically.

Here are the pertinent facts

Muscles unless adequately exercised or used will become weak and inefficient. Let's take a look at some of the evidence which shows why regular vigorous exercise is so essential to physical well-being.

Weak back muscles are associated, in many cases, with lower back pain. It has been estimated that 90 % of these backaches may be eliminated by increasing the strength of the back muscles through exercise.

A bulging, sagging abdomen resulting from weakened abdominal muscles is detrimental to good posture.

The efficiency and capacity of your heart, lungs and other organs can be improved by **regular vigourous** exercise.

A fit person is less susceptible to common injuries, and, if injured, recovers more rapidly.

The incidence of degenerative heart diseases may be greater in those who have not followed a physically active life.

Regular vigorous exercise plays an important role in controlling your weight.

Regular vigorous physical activity can help you to reduce emotional and nervous tension.

You are never too old to begin and follow a regular exercise program.

You can collect valuable dividends of physical efficiency from your daily activities

Hidden in the simple activities we do every day are wonderful opportunities to get exercise and keep refreshed. Because we have developed an attitude of "doing it the easy way" we take short-cuts which seldom save time. Consequently we have developed habits to avoid physical exertion.

Here are some routine activities which can be turned into small challenges that will help to maintain physical fitness once you have attained the suggested level of physical capacity for you. Make them a HABIT!

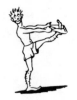

Balance on one foot without support while putting on your socks or shoes.

Give yourself a vigorous rub-down with a rough towel after a shower.

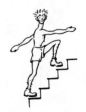

Take the stairs two at a time instead of trudging up one at a time. Avoid elevators for short trips.

Lift your chair, don't shove it.
Bend your knees fully and keep back straight when picking an object off the floor.

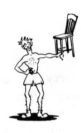

Welcome an opportunity to walk; look for ways you can walk a few blocks rather than ways in which to avoid walking. Step out smartly and breathe deeply.

PHYSICAL FITNESS

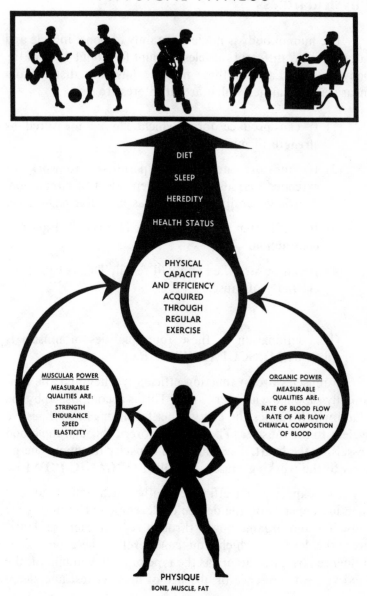

DIET
SLEEP
HEREDITY
HEALTH STATUS

PHYSICAL CAPACITY AND EFFICIENCY ACQUIRED THROUGH REGULAR EXERCISE

MUSCULAR POWER
MEASURABLE QUALITIES ARE:
STRENGTH
ENDURANCE
SPEED
ELASTICITY

ORGANIC POWER
MEASURABLE QUALITIES ARE:
RATE OF BLOOD FLOW
RATE OF AIR FLOW
CHEMICAL COMPOSITION OF BLOOD

PHYSIQUE
BONE, MUSCLE, FAT

Physical fitness

The human body is made up mainly of bone, muscle and fat. Some 639 different muscles account for about 45 % of the body weight. Each of these muscles has four distinct and measurable qualities which are of interest to us.

(1) It can produce force which can be measured as **strength** of muscle.

(2) It can store energy which permits it to work for extended periods of time independent of circulation. This is generally referred to as **muscular endurance.**

(3) It can shorten at varying rates. This is called **speed of contraction.**

(4) It can be stretched and will recoil. This is called the **elasticity** of muscle.

The combination of these four qualities of muscle is referred to as **MUSCULAR POWER.**

If muscles are to function efficiently, they must be continually supplied with energy fuel. This is accomplished by the blood which carries the energy fuel from lungs and digestive system to the muscles. The blood is forced through the blood vessels by the heart. The combined capacity to supply energy fuels to the working muscles is called **ORGANIC POWER.**

The capacity and efficiency with which your body can function depends on the degree of development of both your muscular and organic power through regular exercise. However, the level to which you can develop these powers is influenced by such factors as the type of body you inherit, the food you eat, presence or absence of disease, rest and sleep.

You are physically fit only when you have adequately developed your muscular and organic power to perform with the highest possible efficiency.

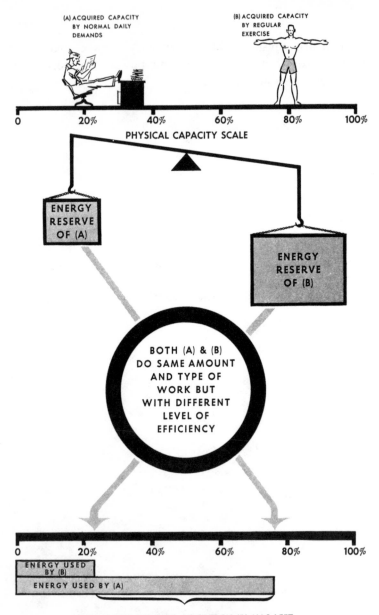

THIS IS THE AMOUNT OF ENERGY (B) HAS LEFT
OVER TO ENJOY HIS RECREATIONAL ACTIVITIES

22

How fit should you be?

Heredity and health determine the top limits to which your physical capacity can be developed. This is known as your potential physical capacity. This potential capacity varies from individual to individual. Most of us for example, could train for a lifetime and never come close to running a four minute mile simply because we weren't "built" for it.

The top level at which you can perform physically **right now** is called your "acquired capacity" because it has been acquired or developed through physical activity in your daily routines.

Your body, like a car, functions most efficiently well below its acquired capacity. A car, for example, driven at its

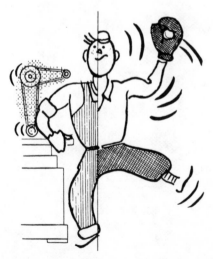

LEAD A BALANCED LIFE

23

top speed of, say, 110 miles per hour uses more gas per mile than when it is driven around 50-60 miles per hour, which is well below its capacity. Your body functions in the same way, in that the ratio of work performed to energy expended is better when it functions well below acquired capacity.

You can avoid wastage of energy by acquiring a level of physical capacity well above the level required to perform your normal daily tasks. This can be accomplished by supplementing your daily physical activity with a balanced exercise program performed regularly. Your capacity increases as you progressively increase the load on your muscular and organic systems.

Exercise will increase physical endurance and stamina thus providing a greater reserve of energy for leisure time activities.

PHYSICAL EFFICIENCY COMPARISONS

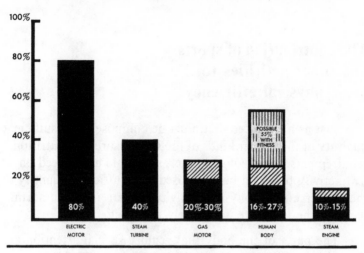

The efficiency of the human body compares poorly with the modern machine.
However, through regular exercise its efficiency can be considerably increased.

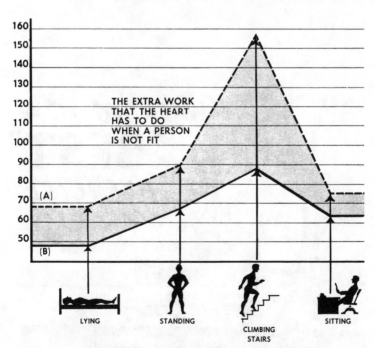

This graph illustrates the number of heart beats required for
your different routine activities by a human being, (A) before
and (B) after a regular vigorous exercise programme.

The contribution of sports and other activities to basic physical efficiency

Just as a balanced diet must be composed of a sufficient quantity of the proper kinds of foods to ensure that nutritional requirements are adequately met, so should a balanced physical activity program be composed of a sufficient quantity of the proper kind of physical activity so that all the important parts of the body are adequately exercised.

The parts of the body that require special attention are the muscles of the shoulder and arms, abdomen and back, legs, and the heart, lungs and blood vessels.

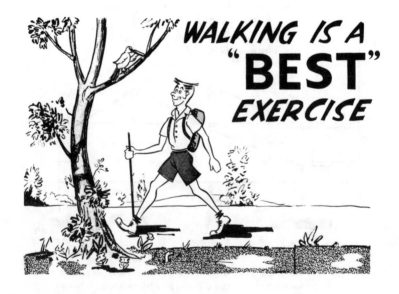

No single sport provides a truly balanced development for all parts of the body. This can only be acquired by regular participation in a number of carefully selected sports. Such participation, however, is not possible for the average person for a number of reasons — availability of play opportunity, time, finances. The most pratical physical fitness scheme for most of us is participation in one or two sports supplemented by a balanced set of exercises. The 5BX program has been designed to bring physical fitness within the reach of any healthy person who is willing to devote 11 minutes a day to a simple but balanced set of exercises.

Common sense about exercise

"It won't do you any good to exercise unless you do it until it hurts" — the saying goes. This is absolutely false. Although you may get some benefit from doing exercises until "it hurts", this is not necessary in order to acquire an adequate level of physical fitness. As a matter of fact, greater benefits can be derived from exercise by avoiding stiffness and soreness.

There are basically two ways in which you can avoid discomfort and still develop high levels of physical capacity:

* Warm up properly before participating in any strenuous physical activity such as sprinting, handball, tennis, etc.

* Start any training program at a low level of activity and work up by easy stages.

Warming up

The 5BX Plan was designed so that no additional warmup is necessary in order to receive its maximum benefits.

The older one is, the more necessary proper warming up becomes to avoid "strained" muscles. The 5BX Plan has a built-in method of warmup. This is achieved in two ways:

— by the arrangement of the exercises; and

— by the manner in which these exercises are performed.

For example, the first exercise is a stretching and loosening exercise which limbers up the large muscles of the body. In addition, this exercise should be started very slowly and easily, with a gradual increase in speed and vigour.

Let us see how this principle applies to exercise No. 1, which requires you to touch the floor. You should not force yourself to do it on the first attempt, but rather start by pushing down very gently and slowly as far as you can without undue strain — then on each succeeding try push down a little harder, and, at the same time, do the exercise a little faster so that by the end of two minutes you are touching the floor and moving at the necessary speed. All the exercises can be performed in this manner.

If you choose to do the exercises in the morning, and are a slowstarter, as soon as the alarm rings, stretch, arch your back, lift your legs, and start riding your bicycle.

Weight control — exercise

When you are overweight, you have more fat stored up in your body than is necessary or good for you.

You become overweight and flabby when you eat more "high-calorie food" than your body can use. Foods such as fats, sugars, starches, etc., supply the energy your body needs for its work. If you eat more high-calorie foods than is required for your daily work the surplus is stored in the form of fat. Fat is stored under the skin and around the internal organs.

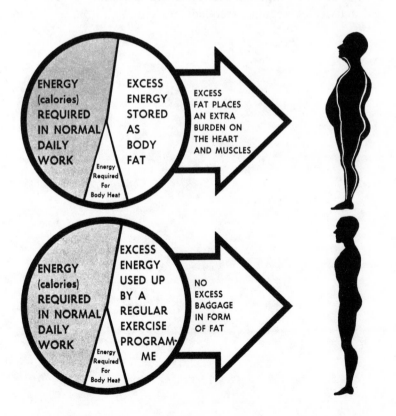

Everyone has, or should have some fat on his body. However, excessive fat storage, particularly about vital organs, impairs physical efficiency and health. Fat makes the heart work harder since each extra pound of body fat requires about one quarter of a mile of blood vessels. It is obvious, therefore, that you cannot acquire the highest level of physical efficiency when you are overweight.

The accumulation of fat on your body can be prevented or reduced either by eating less high-calorie foods or increasing your physical activity. It is better still to combine these two by cutting down on high-calorie foods and increasing your physical activity by regular, frequent exercise.

What is it?

The 5BX Plan is composed of 6 charts arranged in progression. Each chart is composed of 5 exercises which are always performed in the same order and in the same maximum time limit, but, as you progress from chart to chart, there are slight changes in each basic exercise with a gradual demand for more effort.

A sample rating scale of **Chart 3** is reproduced on the next page and is to be used in the following way:

LEVEL

These are the Physical Capacity levels, each indicated by a letter of the alphabet.

EXERCISES

Exercises 1, 2, 3 and 4 apply to the first four exercises described and illustrated on the following pages. The column headed 1 represents exercise 1 (toe touch), etc. The figures in each column indicate the number of times that each exercise is to be repeated in the time allotted for that exercise. Exercise 5 is running on the spot. Two activities may be substituted for it however, and if you prefer, you may run or walk the recommended distance in the required time in place of the stationary run of exercise 5.

MINUTES FOR EACH EXERCISE

The allotted time for each exercise is noted here. These times remain the same throughout all the charts. Total time for exercises 1 through 5 is 11 minutes.

PHYSICAL CAPACITY RATING SCALE

Level	EXERCISE					1 mile run	2 mile walk
	1	2	3	4	5	In minutes	
A+	30	32	47	24	550	8	25
A	30	31	45	22	540	8	25
A−	30	30	43	21	525	8	25
B+	28	28	41	20	510	$8\frac{1}{4}$	26
B	28	27	39	19	500	$8\frac{1}{4}$	26
B−	28	26	37	18	490	$8\frac{1}{4}$	26
C+	26	25	35	17	480	$8\frac{1}{2}$	27
C	26	24	34	17	465	$8\frac{1}{2}$	27
C−	26	23	33	16	450	$8\frac{1}{2}$	27
D+	24	22	31	15	430	$8\frac{3}{4}$	28
D	24	21	30	15	415	$8\frac{3}{4}$	28
D−	24	20	29	15	400	$8\frac{3}{4}$	29
Minutes for each exercise	2	1	1	1	6		

AGE GROUPS

12 yrs   maintains D+
13 yrs   maintains C+
14 yrs   maintains B+
35-39 yrs maintains B
40-44 yrs maintains C

FLYING CREW

40-44 yrs maintains A+
45-49 yrs maintains B

NOTE:

It is important that the exercises at any level be completed in 11 minutes. However, it is likely that in the early stages, an individual will complete certain exercises in less than the allotted time while others may require longer. In these circumstances the times allotted for individual exercises may be varied within the total 11 minute period.

HOW FAR SHOULD YOU PROGRESS?

The level of Physical Capacity to which you should progress is determined by your "Age Group". Levels for "Flying Crew" are listed separately. See "Your Physical Capacity Level" on page 32.

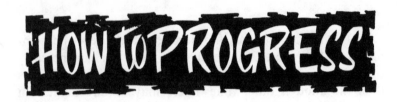

HOW to PROGRESS

Check your daily schedule and determine the time most convenient for you to do the exercises. It should be the same time each day.

Here are some suggested times:

— before breakfast;

— late morning or afternoon, at your place of employment;

— after your regular recreational period;

— in the evening just before you retire.

Regardless of the time you choose **START TODAY.**

Maximum Rate of Progression Through Chart 1 According to Age

> 20 years or under, at least 1 day at each level
>
> 20-29 years, at least 2 days at each level
>
> 30-39 years, at least 4 days at each level
>
> 40-49 years, at least 7 days at each level
>
> 50-59 years, at least 8 days at each level
>
> 60 years and over, at least 10 days at each level

(If you feel stiff or sore, or if you are unduly breathless at any time, ease up and slow down your rate of progression. This is particularly applicable to the older age groups.)

A note of caution

Even if you feel able to start at a high level and progress at a faster rate than indicated — DON'T DO IT — Start at the bottom of chart 1 and work up from level to level as recommended.

For best results from 5BX the exercises must be done *regularly*. Remember, it may take you 6, 8, 10 months or more of daily exercises to attain the level recommended for you, but once you have attained it, only 3 periods of exercise per week will maintain this level of physical capacity.

If for any reason (illness, etc.) you stop doing 5BX regularly and you wish to begin again, *do not* recommence at the level you had attained previously.

Do drop back several levels — until you find one you can do without undue strain. After a period of inactivity of longer than two months, or one month if caused by illness, it is recommended that you start again at Chart 1.

HOW to PROGRESS

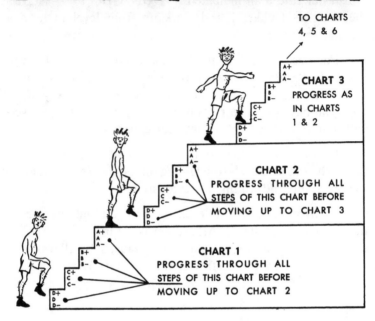

TO CHARTS
4, 5 & 6

CHART 3
PROGRESS AS
IN CHARTS
1 & 2

CHART 2
PROGRESS THROUGH ALL
STEPS OF THIS CHART BEFORE
MOVING UP TO CHART 3

CHART 1
PROGRESS THROUGH ALL
STEPS OF THIS CHART BEFORE
MOVING UP TO CHART 2

MAKE 5BX A HABIT

Start at the lowest Physical Capacity Level of Chart 1
(D—). Repeat each exercise in the allotted time or do the 5
exercises in 11 minutes. Move upward on the same chart to the
next level (D) only after you can complete all the required
movements at your present level within 11 minutes. Continue
to progress upward in this manner until you can complete all
the required movements at level A+ within 11 minutes. Now
start at the bottom of Chart 2 (D—), and continue in this
fashion upwards through the levels, and from chart to chart
until you reach the level for your age group, i.e., age 35-39 (B
Chart 3) does 32 levels from D— on Chart 1 to B on Chart 3.

CHART 1

PHYSICAL CAPACITY RATING SCALE

Level	EXERCISE					½ mile run	1 mile walk
	1	2	3	4	5	In minutes	
A+	20	18	18	13	400	5½	17
A	18	17	17	12	375	5½	17
A−	16	15	16	11	335	5½	17
B+	14	13	15	9	320	6	18
B	12	12	14	8	305	6	18
B−	10	11	13	7	280	6	18
C+	8	9	12	6	260	6½	19
C	7	8	10	5	235	6½	19
C−	6	7	8	4	205	6½	19
D+	4	5	6	3	175	7	20
D	3	4	5	3	145	7½	21
D−	2	3	4	2	100	8	21
Minutes for each exercise	2	1	1	1	6		

AGE GROUPS

6 yrs maintains B
7 yrs maintains A

Exercise I

Feet astride, arms upward.

— Forward bend to floor touching then stretch upward and backward bend.

— Do not strain to keep knees straight.

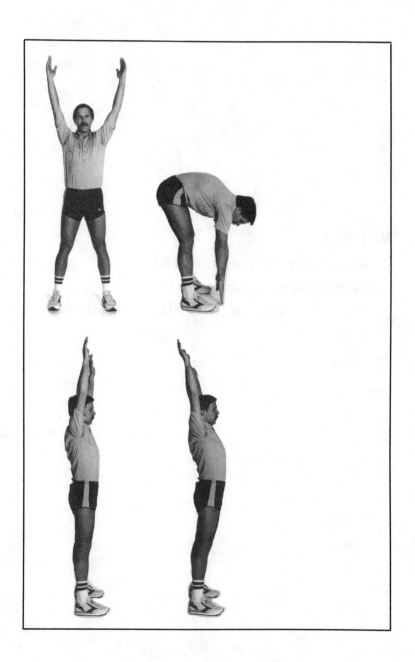

Exercise II

Back lying, feet 6" apart, arms at sides.

— Sit up just far enough to see your heels.

— Keep legs straight, head and shoulders must clear the floor.

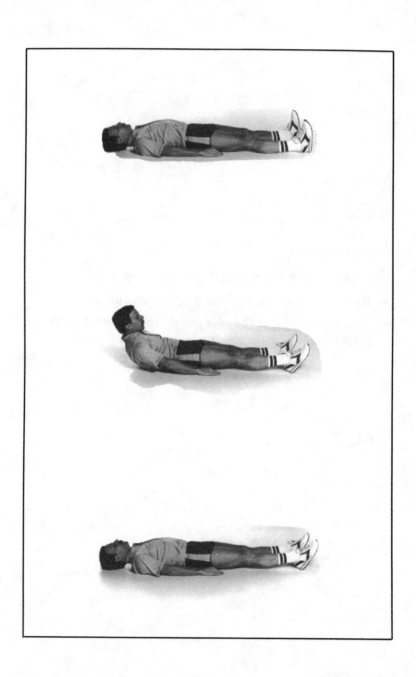

Exercise III

Front lying, palms placed under the thighs.

— Raise head and one leg, repeat using legs alternately.
— Keep leg straight at the knee, thighs must clear the palms.
(Count one each time second leg touches floor.)

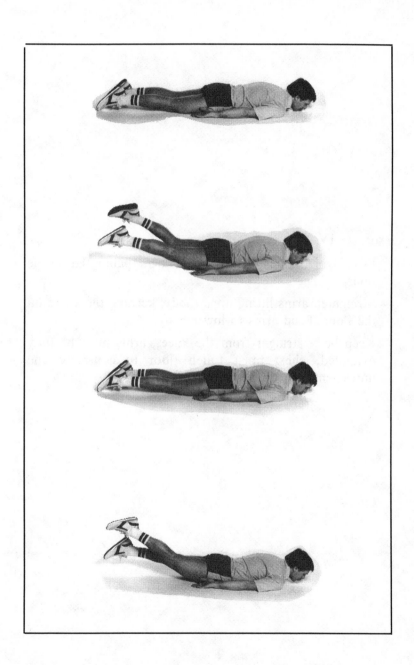

Exercise IV

Front lying, hands under the shoulders, palms flat on the floor.

— Straighten arms lifting upper body, keeping the knees on the floor. Bend arms to lower body.

— Keep body straight from the knees, arms must be fully extended, chest must touch floor to complete one movement.

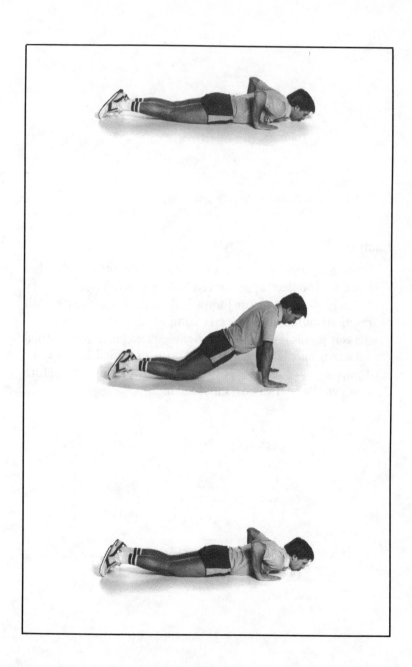

Exercise V

Stationary run — (count a step each time left foot touches floor — Lift feet approximately 4 inches off floor). Every 75 steps do 10 "scissor jumps". Repeat this sequence until required number of steps is completed.

Scissor jumps — Stand with right leg and left arm extended forward, and left leg and right arm extended backward. Jump up — change position of arms and legs before landing. Repeat (arms shoulder high).

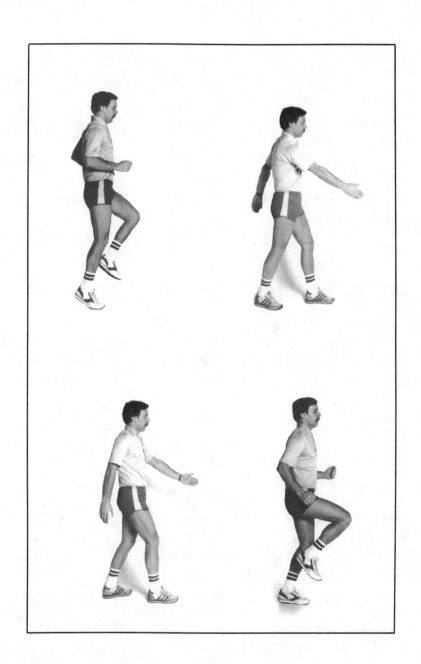

CHART 2

Level	EXERCISE					1 mile run	2 mile walk
	1	2	3	4	5	In minutes	
A+	30	23	33	20	500	9	30
A	29	21	31	19	485	9	31
A−	28	20	29	18	470	9	32
B+	26	18	27	17	455	9½	33
B	24	17	25	16	445	9½	33
B−	22	16	23	15	440	9½	33
C+	20	15	21	14	425	10	34
C	19	14	19	13	410	10	34
C−	18	13	17	12	395	10	34
D+	16	12	15	11	380	10½	35
D	15	11	14	10	360	10½	35
D−	14	10	13	9	335	10½	35
Minutes for each exercise	2	1	1	1	6		

AGE GROUPS

8 yrs	maintains D−
9 yrs	maintains C−
10 yrs	maintains B−
11 yrs	maintains A−
45-49 yrs	maintains A+
50-60 yrs	maintains C+

49

Exercise I

Feet astride, arms upward.

— Touch floor and press (bounce) once then stretch upward and backward bend. Do not strain to keep knees straight.

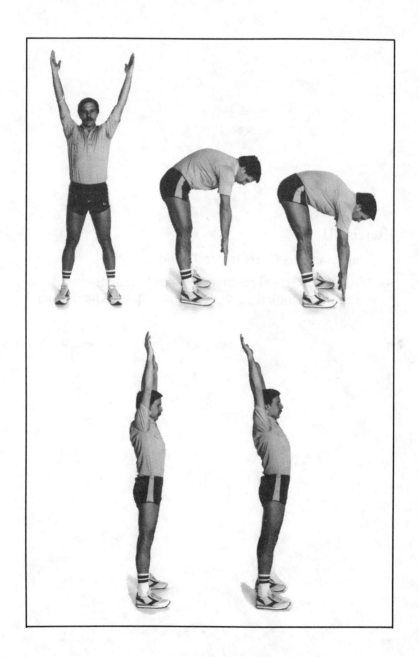

Exercise II

Back lying, feet 6" apart, arms at sides.

— "Sit up" to vertical position, keep feet on floor even if it is necessary to hook them under a chair. Allow knees to bend slightly.

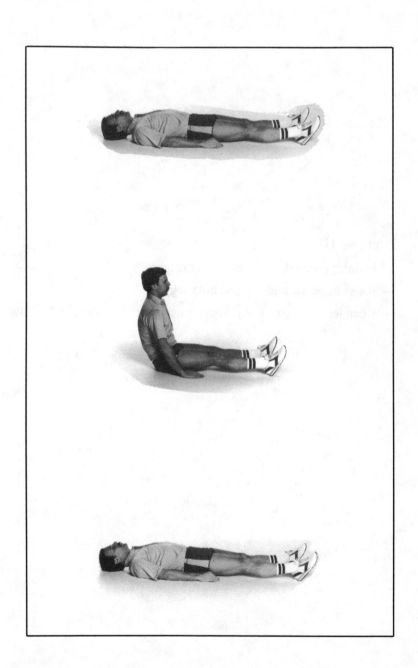

Exercise III

Front lying, palms placed under thighs.

— Raise head, shoulders, and both legs.

— Keep legs straight, both thighs must clear the palms.

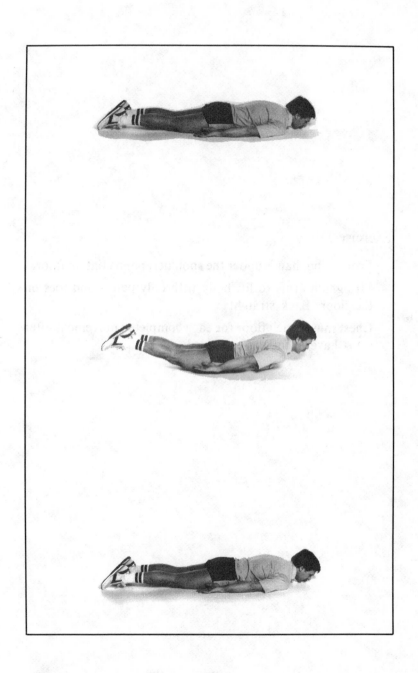

Exercise IV

Front lying, hands under the shoulder, palms flat on floor.

— Straighten arms to lift body with only palms and toes on the floor. Back straight.

— Chest must touch floor for each completed movement after arms have been fully extended.

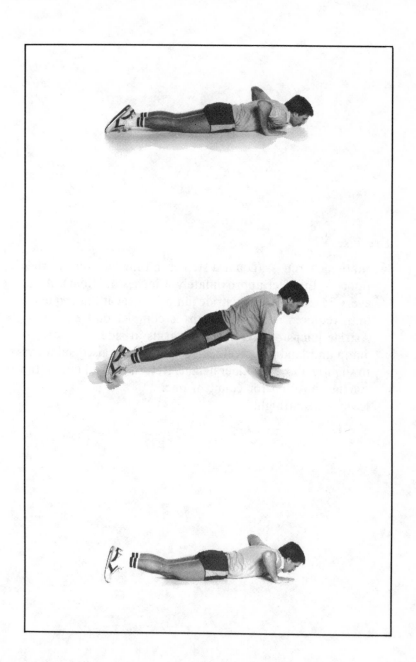

Exercise V

Stationary run — (count a step each time left foot touches floor — Lift feet approximately 4 inches off floor). After every 75 steps, do 10 "astride jumps". Repeat this sequence until required number of steps is completed.

Astride jumps — feet together, arms at side.

Jump and land with feet astride and arms raised sideways to slightly above shoulder height. Return with a jump to the starting position for count of one.

Keep arms straight.

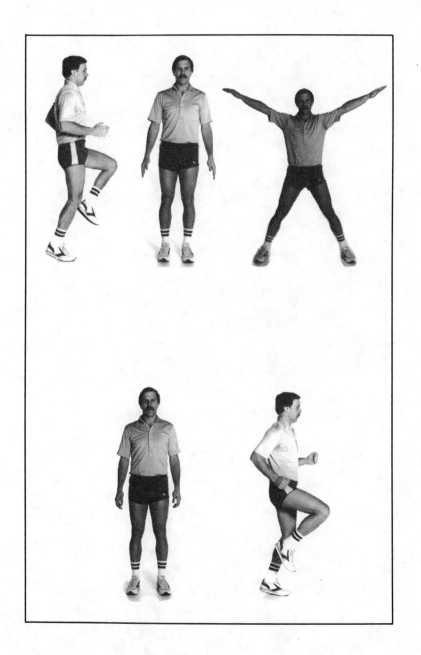

CHART 3

PHYSICAL CAPACITY RATING SCALE

Level	EXERCISE					1 mile run	2 mile walk
	1	2	3	4	5	In minutes	
A+	30	32	47	24	550	8	25
A	30	31	45	22	540	8	25
A−	30	30	43	21	525	8	25
B+	28	28	41	20	510	$8\frac{1}{4}$	26
B	28	27	39	19	500	$8\frac{1}{4}$	26
B−	28	26	37	18	490	$8\frac{1}{4}$	26
C+	26	25	35	17	480	$8\frac{1}{2}$	27
C	26	24	34	17	465	$8\frac{1}{2}$	27
C−	26	23	33	16	450	$8\frac{1}{2}$	27
D+	24	22	31	15	430	$8\frac{3}{4}$	28
D	24	21	30	15	415	$8\frac{3}{4}$	28
D−	24	20	29	15	400	$8\frac{3}{4}$	29
Minutes for each exercise	2	1	1	1	6		

AGE GROUPS

12 yrs   maintains D+
13 yrs   maintains C+
14 yrs   maintains B+
35-39 yrs maintains B
40-44 yrs maintains C

FLYING CREW

40-44 yrs maintains A+
45-49 yrs maintains B

Exercise I

Feet astride, arms upward.

— Touch floor 6" outside left foot, again between feet and press once then 6" outside right foot, bend backward as far as possible, repeat, reverse direction after half the number of counts. Do not strain to keep knees straight, return to erect position.

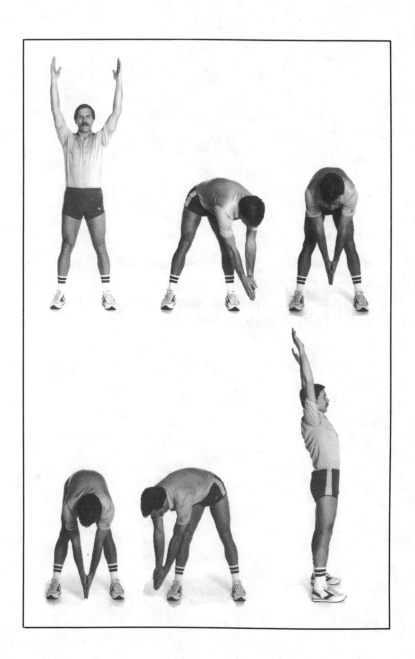

Exercise II

Back lying, feet 6" apart, arms clasped behind head. Allow knees to bend slightly.

— Sit up to vertical position, keep feet on floor, hook feet under chair, etc., only if necessary.

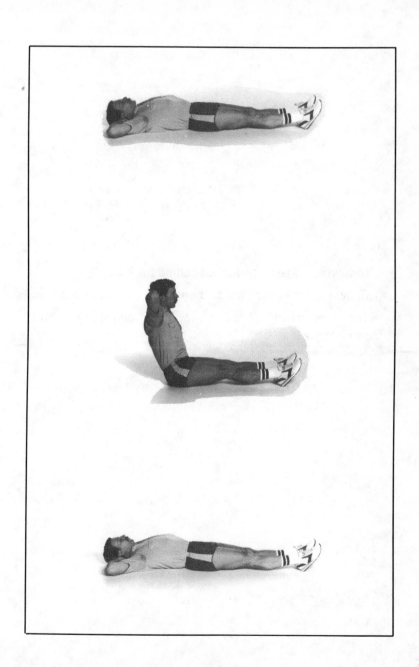

Exercise III

Front lying, hands interlocked behind the back.

— Lift head, shoulders, chest and both legs as high as possible.

— Keep legs straight, and raise chest and both thighs completely off floor.

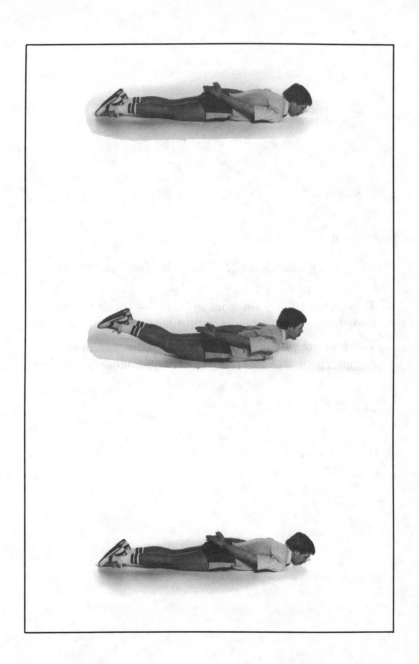

Exercise IV

Front lying, hands under the shoulders, palms flat on floor.

— Touch chin to floor in front of hands — touch forehead to floor behind hands before returning to up position.

— There are three definite movements, chin, forehead, arms straightened. DO NOT do in one continuous movement.

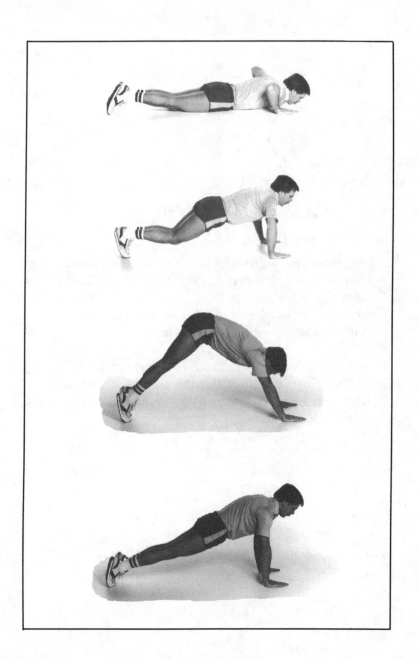

Exercise V

Stationary run — (count a step each time left foot touches floor — Lift feet approximately 4 inches off floor). After every 75 steps do 10 "half knee bends". Repeat this sequence until required number of steps is completed.

Half knee bends — Feet together, hands on hips, knees bent to form an angle of about 110 degrees. Do not bend knees past a right angle. Straighten to upright position, raising heel off floor, return to starting position each time.

Keep feet in contact with floor — the back upright and straight at all times.

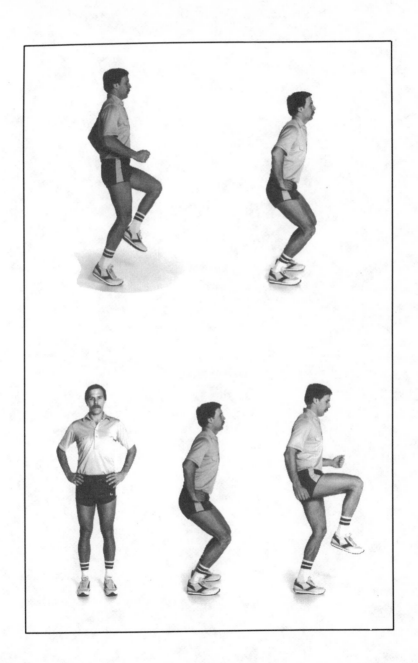

CHART 4

PHYSICAL CAPACITY RATING SCALE

Level	EXERCISE					1 mile run	2 mile walk
	1	2	3	4	5	In minutes	
A+	30	22	50	42	400	7	19
A	30	22	49	40	395	7	19
A−	30	22	49	37	390	7	19
B+	28	21	47	34	380	$7\frac{1}{4}$	20
B	28	21	46	32	375	$7\frac{1}{4}$	20
B−	28	21	46	30	365	$7\frac{1}{4}$	20
C+	26	19	44	28	355	$7\frac{1}{2}$	21
C	26	19	43	26	345	$7\frac{1}{2}$	21
C−	26	19	43	24	335	$7\frac{1}{2}$	21
D+	24	18	41	21	325	$7\frac{3}{4}$	23
D	24	18	40	19	315	$7\frac{3}{4}$	23
D−	24	18	40	17	300	$7\frac{3}{4}$	23
Minutes for each exercise	2	1	1	1	6		

AGE GROUPS

15 yrs   maintains D−
16-17 yrs maintains C+
25-29 yrs maintains A+
30-34 yrs maintains C−

FLYING CREW

30-34 yrs maintains B
35-39 yrs maintains C−

Exercise I

Feet astride, arms upward.

— Touch floor outside left foot, between feet, press once then outside right foot, circle bend backwards as far as possible, reverse direction after half the number of counts. Do not strain to keep knees straight.

— Keep arms above head and make full circle, bending backward past vertical each time.

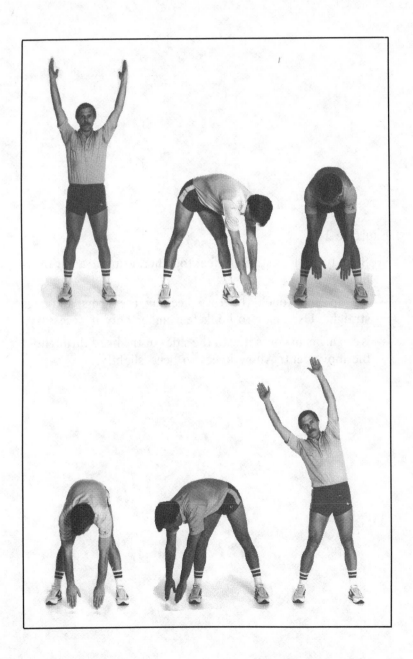

Exercice II

Back lying, legs straight, feet together, arms straight overhead.

— Sit up and touch the toes keeping the arms and legs straight. Use chair to hook feet under only if necessary.

— Keep arms in contact with the sides of the head throughout the movement. Allow knees to bend slightly.

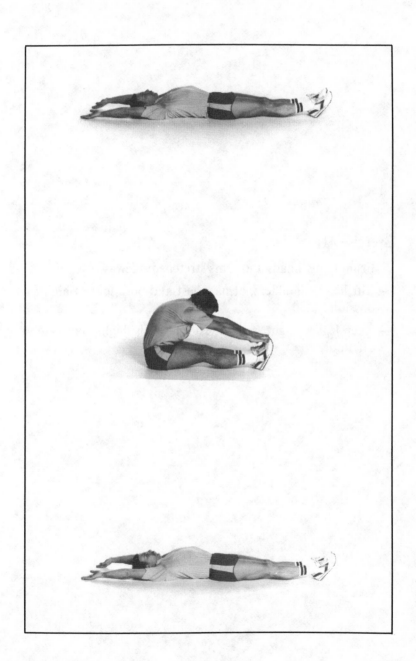

Exercise III

Front lying, hands and arms stretched sideways.

— Lift head, shoulders, arms, chest and both legs as high as possible.

— Keep legs straight, raise chest and both thighs completely off floor.

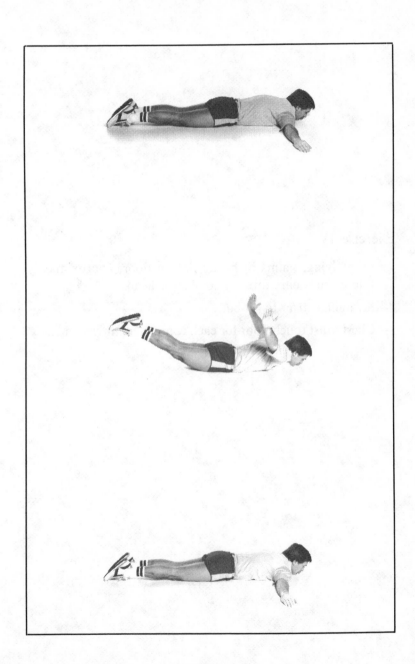

Exercise IV

Front lying, palms of hands flat on floor, approximately 1 foot from ears directly to side of head.

— Straighten arms to lift body.

— Chest must touch floor for each completed movement.

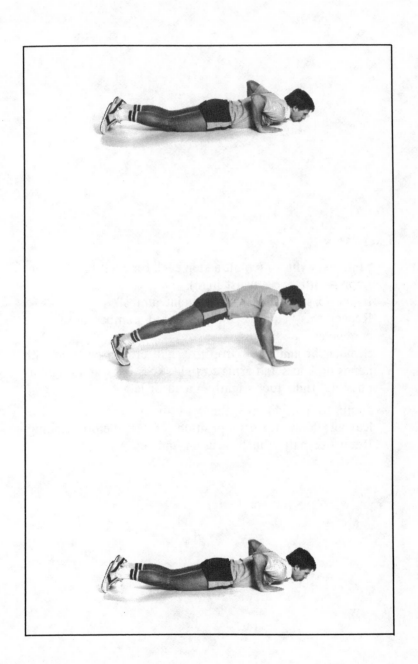

Exercise V

Stationary run — (count a step each time left foot touches floor — lift knees waist high).
Every 75 steps do 10 "semi-squat jumps".
Repeat this sequence until required number of steps is completed.
Semi-squat jumps — Drop to a half crouch position with hands on knees and arms straight, keep back as straight as possible, right foot slightly ahead of left.

— Jump to upright position with body straight and feet leaving floor. Reverse position of feet before landing. Return to half crouch position and repeat.

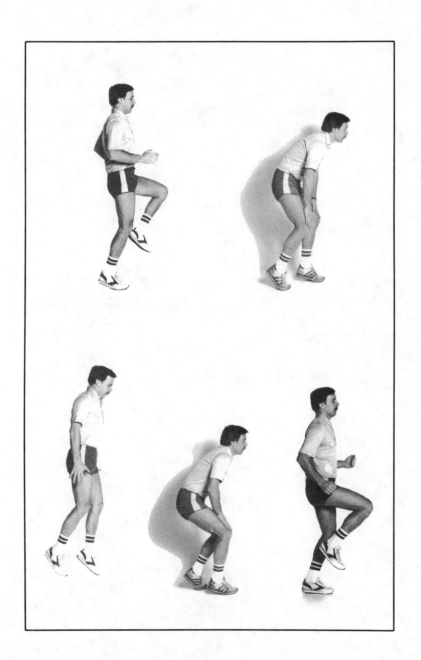

CHART 5

Level	EXERCISE					1 mile run
	1	2	3	4	5	Mins : Secs
A+	30	40	50	44	500	6 : 00
A	30	39	49	43	485	6 : 06
A−	30	38	48	42	475	6 : 09
B+	28	36	47	40	465	6 : 12
B	28	35	46	39	455	6 : 15
B−	28	34	45	38	445	6 : 21
C+	26	32	44	36	435	6 : 27
C	26	31	43	35	420	6 : 33
C−	26	30	42	34	410	6 : 39
D+	24	28	41	32	400	6 : 45
D	24	27	40	31	385	6 : 51
D−	24	26	39	30	375	7 : 00
Minutes for each exercise	2	1	1	1	6	

AGE GROUPS

18-25 yrs maintains C

FLYING CREW

Under 25 yrs maintains B+

25-29 yrs maintains D+

85

Exercise I

Feet astride, arms upward, hands clasped, arms straight.

— Touch floor outside left foot, between feet, press once then outside right foot, circle bend backwards as far as possible. Reverse direction after half the number of counts. Do not strain to keep knees straight.

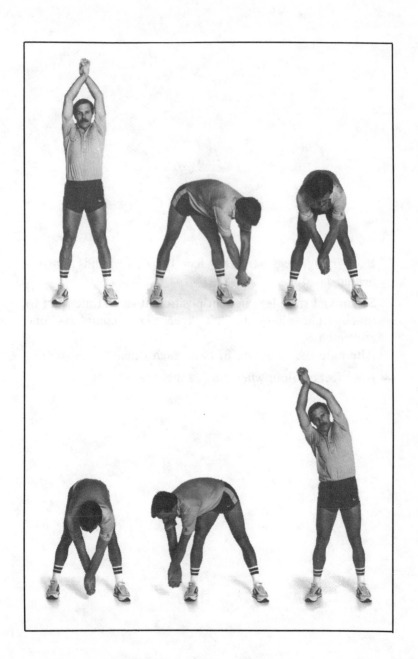

Exercise II

Back lying, legs straight, feet together, hands clasped behind head.

— Sit up and raise legs in bent position at same time twist to touch right elbow to left knee. This completes one movement.
Alternate the direction of twist each time.

— Keep feet off floor when elbow touches knee.

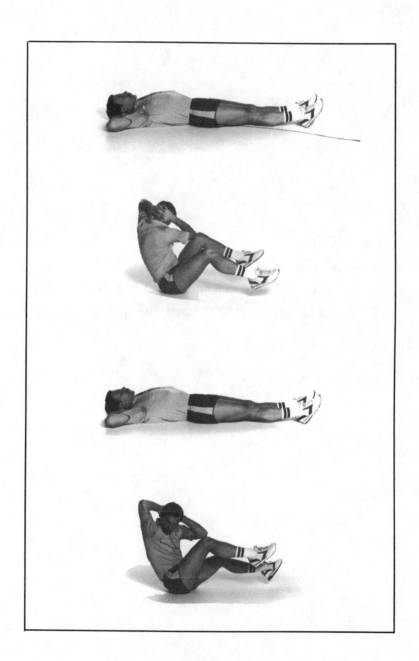

Exercise III

Front lying, arms extended overhead.

— Raise arms, head, chest and both legs as high as possible.

— Keep legs and arms straight, chest and both thighs completely off floor.

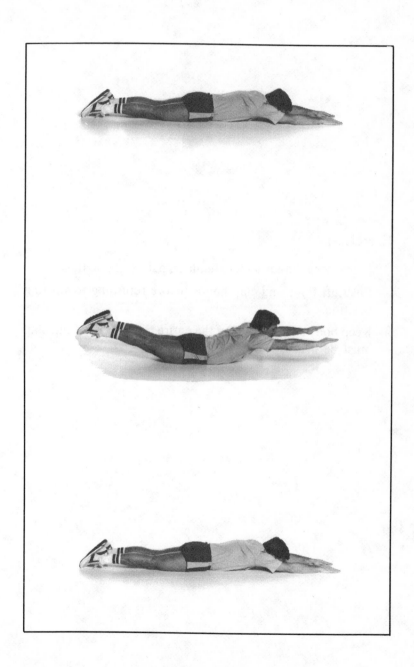

Exercise IV

Front lying, hands under shoulder, palms flat on floor.

— Push off floor and clap hands before returning to starting position.

— Keep body straight during the entire movement. Hand clap must be heard.

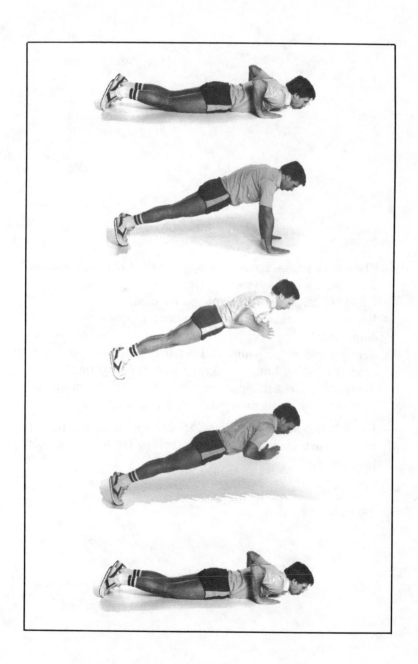

Exercise V

Stationary run — (count a step each time left foot touches floor — lift knees waist high).
Every 75 steps do 10 "semi-spread eagle jumps".
Repeat this sequence until required number of steps is completed.
Semi-spread eagle jumps — Feet together, drop to a half crouch position hands on knees with arms straight.
Jump up to feet astride swing arms overhead in mid-air, return directly to starting position on landing.

— Raise hands above head level, spread feet at least shoulder width apart in astride position before landing with feet together.

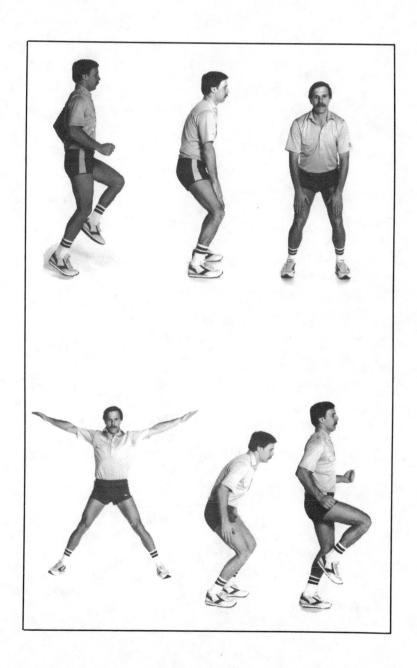

CHART 6

Level	EXERCISE					1 mile run
	1	2	3	4	5	Mins : Secs
A+	30	50	40	40	600	5 : 00
A	30	48	39	39	580	5 : 03
A−	30	47	38	38	555	5 : 09
B+	28	45	37	36	530	5 : 12
B	28	44	36	35	525	5 : 18
B−	28	43	35	34	515	5 : 24
C+	26	41	34	32	505	5 : 27
C	26	40	33	31	495	5 : 33
C−	26	39	32	30	485	5 : 39
D+	24	37	31	28	475	5 : 45
D	24	36	30	27	460	5 : 51
D−	24	35	29	26	450	6 : 00
Minutes for each exercise	2	1	1	1	6	

PHYSICAL CAPACITIES IN THIS
CHART ARE USUALLY FOUND
ONLY IN CHAMPION ATHLETES.

Exercise I

Feet astride, arms upward, hands reverse clasped, arms straight.

— Touch floor outside left foot, between feet, press once then outside right foot, circle bend backwards as far as possible. Reverse direction after half the number of counts.

— Keep hands tightly reverse clasped at all times.

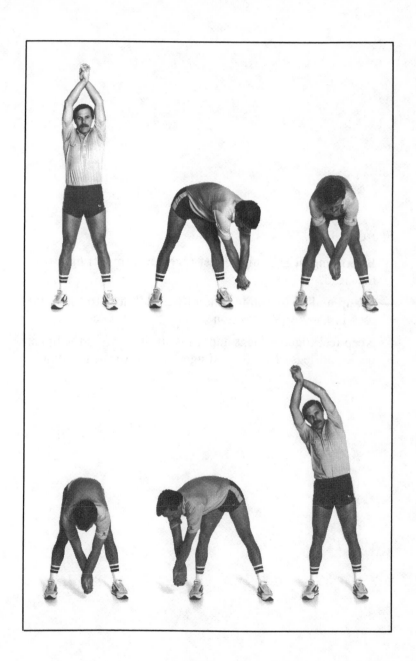

Exercise II

Back lying, legs straight, feet together, arms straight over the head.

— Sit up and at the same time lifting both legs to touch the toes in a pike (V) position.

— Keep feet together, legs and arms straight, all of the upper back and legs clear floor, fingers touch toes each time.

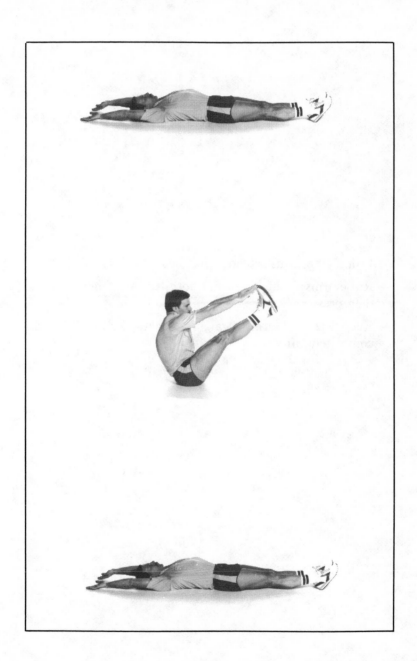

Exercise III

Front lying, arms extended over head.

— Raise arms, head, chest and both legs as high as possible then press back once.

— Keep legs and arms straight — chest and both thighs completely off floor.

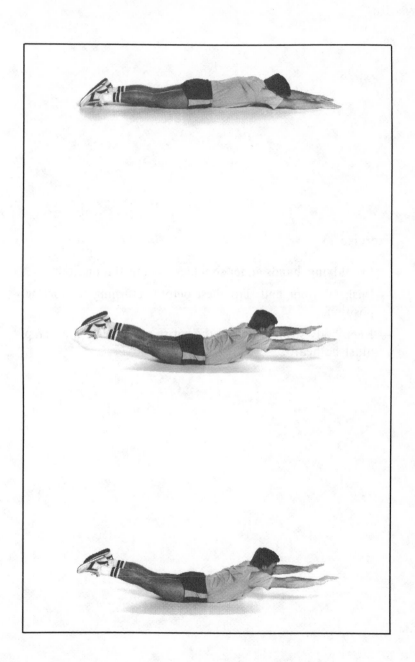

Exercise IV

Front lying, hands under shoulders, palms flat on floor.

— Push off floor and slap chest before returning to starting position.

— Keep body straight during the entire movement, chest slap must be heard.

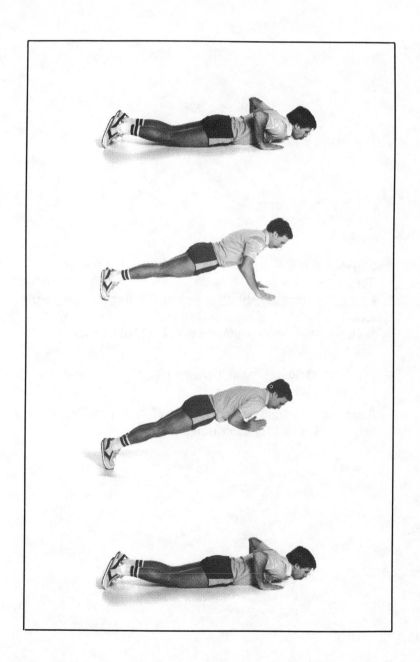

Exercice V

Stationary run — (count a step each time left foot touches floor — lift knees waist high).
Every 75 steps do 10 "jack jumps". Repeat this until required number of steps is completed.
Jack jumps — Feet together, knees bent, sit on heels, finger tips touch floor.

— Jump up, raise legs waist high, keep legs straight and touch toes in midair.

— Keep legs straight, raise feet level to "standing waist height". Touch toes each time.

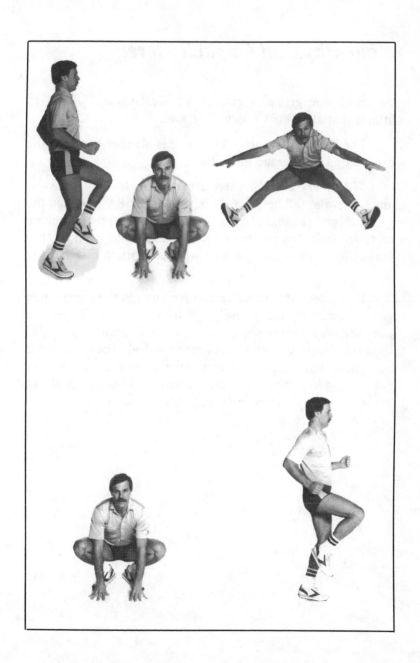

Your Physical Capacity level

Each age group is given a Physical Capacity level to attain; that is, a goal which they should try to reach.

The Physical Capacity levels in this plan are based on the expectation of average individuals.

With every average, there are individuals who surpass it, and those who fall below it. In terms of the 5BX Plan and the goals, this means that there will be some men who are capable of progressing beyond the level indicated, and on the other hand, there will be persons who will never attain this average level.

If you feel able to move further through the charts than your Physical Capacity level, by all means do so. If, on the contrary, you experience great difficulty in approaching this level you should stop at a level which you feel to be within your capability. It is impossible to predict accurately, a level for each individual who uses this program. Use the goals as guides, and apply them with common sense.

Here are a few tips

When you start, defeat the first desire to skip a day; then defeat all such desires as they occur. This exercise program has plenty of bite; the longer you do it the more you will enjoy it.

As you progress well into the program you may find certain levels almost impossible to complete in 11 minutes — work hard at that level — it may take some days or even weeks — then suddenly you will find yourself sailing ahead again.

Counting the steps in exercise 5 can be difficult. You can lose count very easily at times. If you have this problem, here is an easy way to overcome it. Divide the total number of steps 75 and note the answer — place a row of buttons, corresponding in required by 75 and note the answer— place a row of buttons, corresponding in number to this answer, on a handy table or chair. Now count off your first 75 steps — do your ten required movements — and move the first button. Repeat until all the buttons have been removed, finishing up with any left over steps.

For diversity, occasionally an exercise from the previous chart may be substituted.

Wishing is not good enough.